BAY LEAF

MARIAN KIM

CONTENTS

MARIAN KIM

1

PROPERTIES

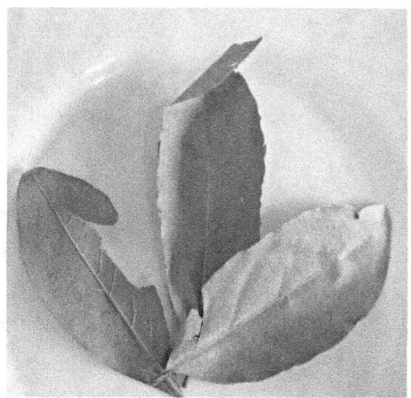

Scientific name: Laurus nobilis

Other names: Bay leaves, laurel leaves, bay tree, sweet laurel, sweet bay, Roman laurel

Properties

Antiseptic (antibacterial, antifungal) properties

Anti-inflammatory properties

Antioxidant which protect the cells from free radical damage

Astringent properties

Diuretic properties (promotes urination)

Diaphoretic properties (promotes sweating)

Appetite stimulating properties

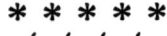

2

USES

Coughs and colds treatment

A compress made with bay leaf infusion can be used to reduce the symptoms of coughs, colds, flus and bronchitis. Warm bay leaf infusions can also be drunk to reduce the symptoms of coughs and colds. The leaves can also be covered with boiling water and the vapor inhaled to help with managing colds. Powdered bay leaves mixed with honey can also be taken to reduce coughing.

Sore throat treatment

Powdered bay leaves can be mixed with water to create a gargle to treat sore throats.

Antipyretic

Bay leaves infusion is used to reduce fevers, promote sweating.

Digestive aid

Infusions made from bay leaves aid digestion. They also relieve flatulence and colic pain. They also stimulate bile flow.

Anorexia treatment

Bay leaves are used to manage anorexia since they can stimulate the appetite.

Diabetes treatment

Some studies have shown that bay leaf reduces blood glucose levels in patients with type 2 diabetes. By so doing it also reduces the risk of developing cardiovascular disease. Powdered bay leaves are used for this function of helping the body process insulin more efficiently and they are usually consumed for 30 days.

Gastric ulcers treatment

Bay leaves are also thought to be useful for the treatment of gastric ulcers.

Cancer treatment

Bay leaves are used to treat cancer.

Migraines treatment

Bay leaves are used to treat migraines and other headaches. Bay leaf infusions can be drunk to relieve the pain. Pastes made from bay leaves can also be applied on the forehead to treat the headache.

Rheumatism treatment

Bay leaves are used to treat rheumatism and joint pains. Poultices made with bay leaves and castor leaves are usually tied around painful joints to reduce the pain and swelling.

Muscle pain treatment

Bay leaves are also used to treat muscle pains.

Insect repellent

Bay leaves have a strong odor and they contain the insect repelling lauric acid. They have been shown by research to be effective for repelling insects like cockroaches.

Lice treatment

Decoctions made from crushed bay leaves are applied to the hair roots for several hours before being rinsed of to get rid of lice.

Insect stings

Bay leaves are also used to treat bee and wasp stings.

Dandruff treatment

Bay leaves are used to treat dandruff.

Amenorrhea treatment

Bay leaves are taken by mouth for amenorrhea since they are thought to induce regular menstruation.

Aiding conception

Bay leaves mixed with anise have been inserted into the vagina to aid conception.

Acting as a contraceptive

A hot water extract of bay leaves is consumed in some places as a contraceptive.

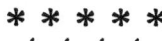

3

SAFETY PRECAUTIONS

Women who are pregnant should avoid eating excessive amounts of bay leaves since some of their chemical compounds can cause miscarriage.

When used for cooking bay leaves should be removed from the dish before serving since they do not soften and they may cut the tongue, injure the digestive system or cause choking.

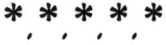

4

DRUG INTERACTIONS

Persons taking medications for diabetes should avoid using bay leaves.

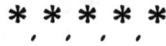

5

COOKING TIPS

Flavor: Sharp

Goes well with: Meat dishes e.g. beef, fish dishes e.g. tuna, rice dishes e.g. pilau and biryani, beans, spiced tea, slow cooking stews, soups and sauces

Can be substituted with: Thyme

Tip: Remove bay leaves from the dish before serving since they do not soften during cooking.

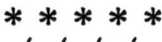

6

HERBAL RECIPES

Bay Leaf Infusion

Equipment

Glass jar with tight fitting lid

***

Ingredients

3 bay leaves

1 cup boiling water

***

Instructions

1. Place the bay leaves in the glass jar and add the boiling water to fill the jar.

2. Close the lid and let the mixture steep for 4 hours to 14 hours (overnight).

3. Strain the herb and the infusion is ready for use.

***

Tips

1. Store the infusion in the refrigerator to lengthen its life.

*****

Bay Leaf Syrup

Equipment

Saucepan

Jar with airtight lid

***

Ingredients

1 quart (1000 ml) filtered water

1 cup bay leaves

1 cup honey

***

Instructions

1. Place the water and bay leaves in a saucepan and bring to a boil.

2. Reduce the heat and let it simmer while it is partially covered until the volume is reduced to half the original volume.

3. Strain the mixture through a sieve or cheesecloth to remove the bay leaves.

4. Measure 1 pint (500 mls) of the liquid and add the honey.

5. Cook for a few minutes as you stir it so that it thickens.

6. Store the syrup in an airtight container in the fridge for up to 2 months.

*****

Bay Leaf Poultice

Equipment

Cheesecloth or old cotton sheet strips

***

Ingredients

1 tablespoon powdered bay leaves

Boiling water

***

Instructions

1. Add enough boiling water to the herb to wet it and make a thick paste.

2. Spoon the herb paste onto the cheesecloth (or bed sheet strips) to make the poultice.

3. To use, apply the poultice to the affected area and cover with another piece of hot, wet cloth. Replace the hot, wet cloth when it cools with another hot one to keep the poultice hot.

*****

Bay Leaf Decoction

Equipment

Non-reactive heavy saucepan

***

Ingredients

1 oz (30 grams) bay leaves

1 pint (500 ml) water

***

Instructions

1. Place the bay leaves and water in the saucepan, cover it and slowly bring the mixture to a simmering boil for 20 minutes.

2. Remove from the heat source and let the mixture cool to drinking temperature.

3. Strain the mixture, measure it and pour the liquid into a clean saucepan.

4. Heat the liquid until it begins to steam. Reduce the heat and let the liquid continue to steam until it is reduced to half its original volume. This may take 45 minutes to 1 hour.

5. Pour the decoction into a clean bottle.

***

Tips

1. Store the decoction in the refrigerator to lengthen its life.

*****

Bay Leaf Tincture

Equipment

Glass jar with tight fitting lid

Dark tincture bottles

Cheesecloth

Labels

***

Ingredients

7 oz (200 gm) of bay leaves

30 oz (1 liter) of 80-100 proof vodka

***

Instructions

1. Fill 1/3 of the glass jar with the chopped bay leaves.

2. Add the vodka to completely fill the jar to the top.

3. Seal the jar and label it with the date of preparation and name of herb used.

4. Store the glass jar in a dark place for 6 weeks ensuring that you shake them weekly.

5. After 6 weeks strain out the herbs with a cheesecloth and pour the tincture into dark tincture bottles.

6. Label the tincture bottles with the date and name of herb used.

7. Store your herbal tinctures away from light and heat.

***

Tips

1. You can leave the herbs in the alcohol for up to 6 months if you want to create very strong tinctures.

*****

Bay Leaf Infused Oil

Equipment

Double boiler

Large glass bowl

Sieve and cheesecloth

Sterilized dark jars

***

Ingredients

16 fl oz. (500 ml) pure vegetable oil such as sweet almond oil or sunflower oil

8 oz. (250 grams) slightly crushed, dry bay leaves

***

Instructions

1. Place the bay leaves and oil in the glass bowl ensuring that the oil covers the herbs. Simmer them in a double boiler for one hour at a temperature of around 120 degrees Fahrenheit (49 degrees Celsius). Do not let the mixture boil. You can repeat this step several times after letting the oils cool to create more concentrated herb infused oils.

2. Strain the mixture through the sieve and cheesecloth into a clean, dark jar ensuring you squeeze out as much oil as you can from the cheesecloth.

3. Label your jars with the manufacturing date, expiry date, herb and oils used.

4. Store your herb infused oils in a cool dark place or in the refrigerator and use them within 3 months.

*****

Bay Leaf Tea

Equipment

Kettle

Tea cup

***

Ingredients

1 teaspoon of finely crushed bay leaves

1 cup of boiling water

Honey to taste (optional)

***

Instructions

1. Put the bay leaves in a tea cup, add the boiling water and let it steep while covered for 10 -15 minutes.

3. Add honey (if using) to suit your taste before drinking.

###

ABOUT THE AUTHOR

Marian Kim is an experienced alternative medicine practitioner.

*****

OTHER BOOKS BY THE AUTHOR

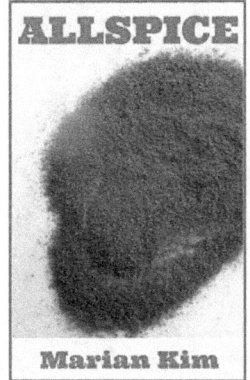

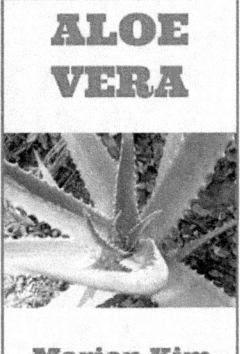

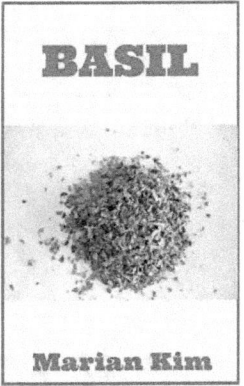

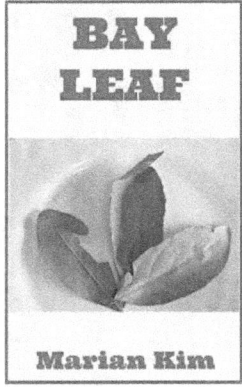

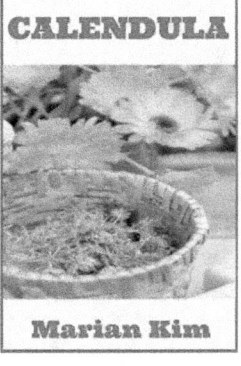

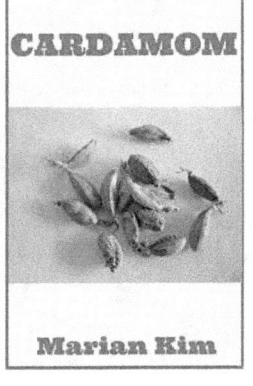

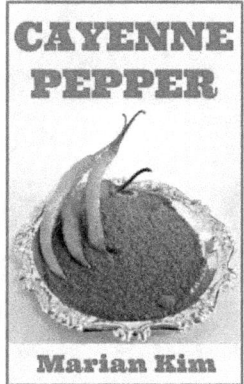

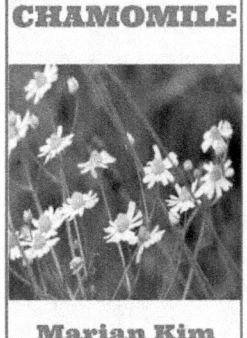

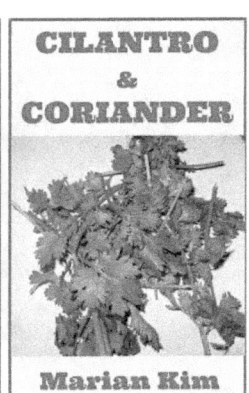

CINNAMON

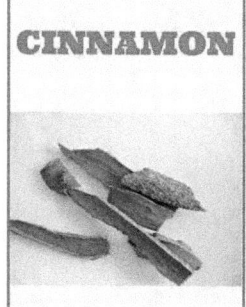

Marian Kim

CLOVES

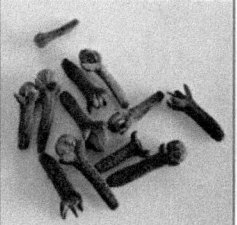

Marian Kim

CUMIN

Marian Kim

DANDELION

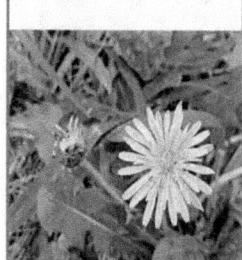

Marian Kim

DILL

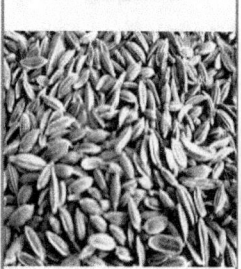

Marian Kim

ECHINACEA

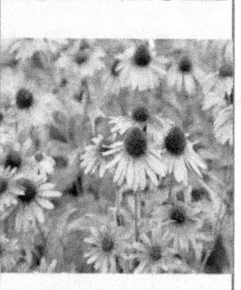

Marian Kim

FENNEL

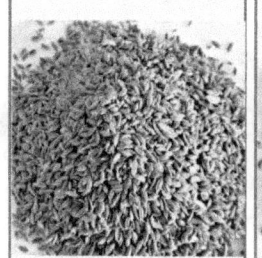

Marian Kim

FENUGREEK

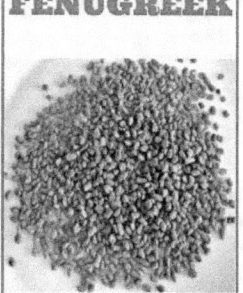

Marian Kim

GARLIC

Marian Kim

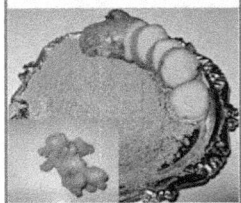
GINGER
Marian Kim

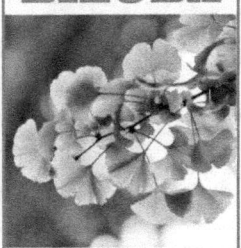
GINKGO BILOBA
Marian Kim

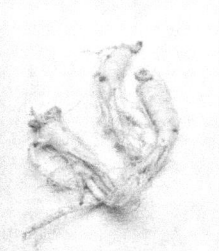
GINSENG
Marian Kim

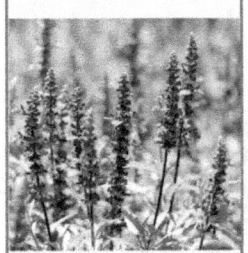
LAVENDER
Marian Kim

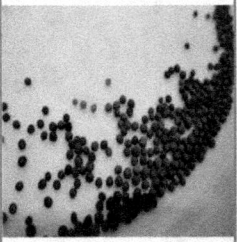
MUSTARD
Marian Kim

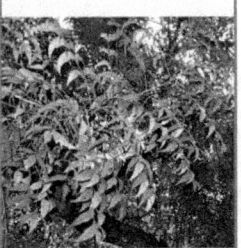
NEEM
Marian Kim

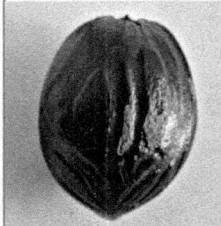
NUTMEG & MACE
Marian Kim

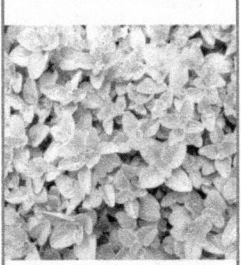
OREGANO
Marian Kim

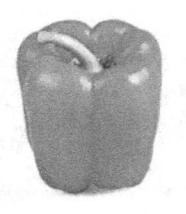
PAPRIKA
Marian Kim

PARSLEY

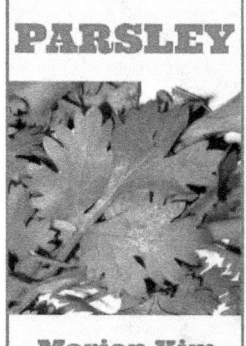

Marian Kim

BLACK & WHITE PEPPER

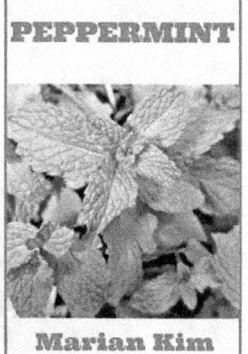

Marian Kim

PEPPERMINT

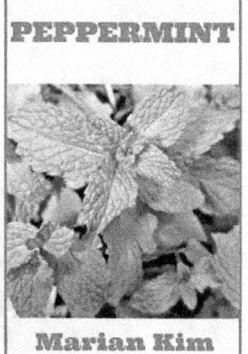

Marian Kim

ROSE HIPS

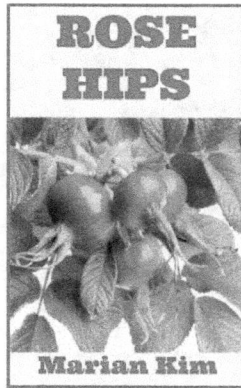

Marian Kim

ROSE PETALS

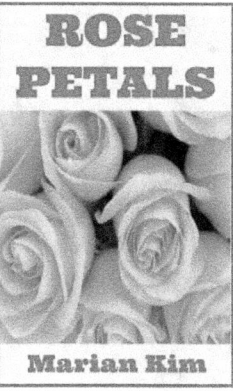

Marian Kim

ROSEMARY

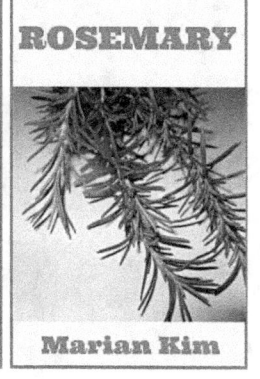

Marian Kim

SAGE

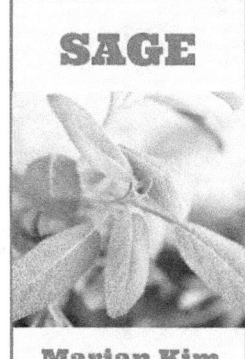

Marian Kim

ST. JOHN'S WORT

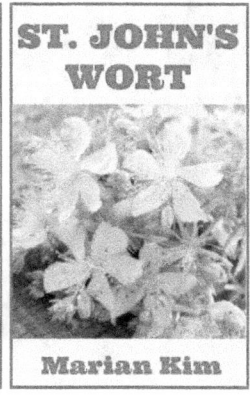

Marian Kim

STAR ANISE

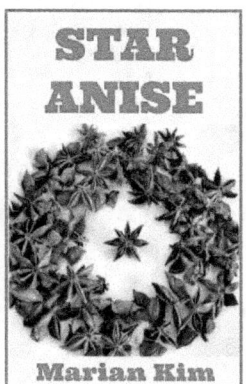

Marian Kim

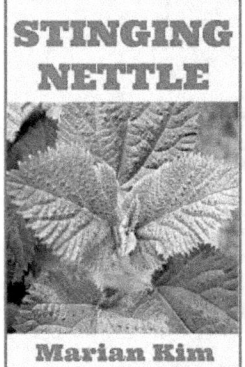

STINGING NETTLE

Marian Kim

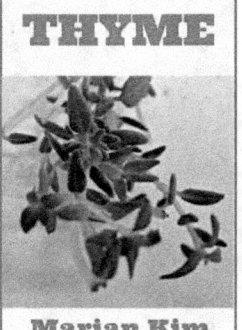

THYME

Marian Kim

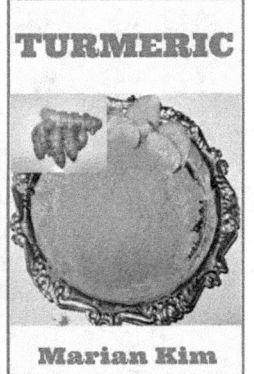

TURMERIC

Marian Kim

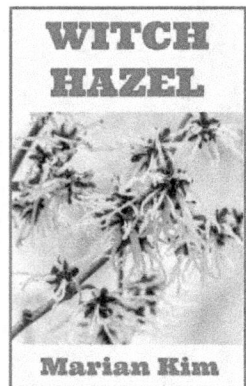

WITCH HAZEL

Marian Kim

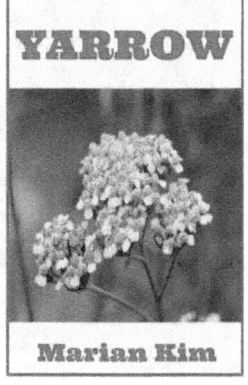

YARROW

Marian Kim

*****